Ruan Silva

Cervical cancer and cytopathology after radiotherapy

Ruan Silva

Cervical cancer and cytopathology after radiotherapy

Follow-up cytopathology in women with cervical cancer after radiotherapy: case series

ScienciaScripts

Imprint
Any brand names and product names mentioned in this book are subject to trademark, brand or patent protection and are trademarks or registered trademarks of their respective holders. The use of brand names, product names, common names, trade names, product descriptions etc. even without a particular marking in this work is in no way to be construed to mean that such names may be regarded as unrestricted in respect of trademark and brand protection legislation and could thus be used by anyone.

Cover image: www.ingimage.com

This book is a translation from the original published under ISBN 978-613-9-64497-1.

Publisher:
Sciencia Scripts
is a trademark of
Dodo Books Indian Ocean Ltd. and OmniScriptum S.R.L publishing group

120 High Road, East Finchley, London, N2 9ED, United Kingdom
Str. Armeneasca 28/1, office 1, Chisinau MD-2012, Republic of Moldova, Europe
Printed at: see last page
ISBN: 978-620-7-74094-9

SUMMARY

Summary

In addition to its role in cervical cancer screening programmes, cytopathology is also an important tool for controlling the effectiveness of treatment in women with cervical cancer, monitoring and detecting residual or recurrent neoplasms or benign reactive changes at an early stage. In this study, we report eight cases of follow-up cytopathology in women with cervical cancer after radiotherapy treatment, assisted by an Oncology Centre in Pernambuco. The main post-treatment cytological findings were described, as well as the histopathological characteristics at diagnosis and the treatments carried out.

Key Words: Radiotherapy; Cytopathology; Cervical cancer; Radiation effects; Morphological changes.

CHAPTER 1

Introduction

Cervical cancer is the third most common cancer in the female population, with an estimated 16,370 new cases in 2018-2019, with a risk of 15.43 per 100,000 women. According to the José Alencar Gomes da Silva National Cancer Institute (INCA), without considering non-melanoma skin tumours, cervical cancer is the first most incident in the North of Brazil (25.62/100,000), the second most frequent in the Northeast (20.47/100,000) and Midwest (18.32/100,000) and ranks fourth in the South (14.07/100,000) and Southeast (9.97/100,000)[(1)] .

Infection with the Human Papillomavirus (HPV) occurs in around 10 to 20 per cent of the sexually active female population between 15 and 49 years of age, and is already well understood to be the main predisposing factor to cervical cancer, being a necessary but not sufficient condition[(2,3)] . Among the risk cofactors involved in cervical carcinogenesis are: sexually transmitted infections, early onset of sexual activity, multiple sexual partners, use of oral contraceptives, smoking, nutritional deficiency and immunological status .[(4)]

The most effective method for the screening, detection and control of cervical cancer is the cytopathological examination, which, if carried out with good coverage and within quality standards, can reduce the incidence rates of invasive cancer by around 90%, being characterised by a simple, low-cost and painless examination that allows the detection of intraepithelial lesions, which can be treated before they become cancer[5,6] .

A large proportion of women are excluded from cancer prevention measures because they are not screened by cervical cancer control programmes due to shyness, fear, lack of information and difficulty in accessing health services, resulting in delays in the diagnosis of intraepithelial lesions and invasive cancer, leading to more aggressive and less effective treatments, as well as increasing mortality rates and hospitalisation costs[7] .

The most widely used clinical and pathological staging for cervical cancer is the FIGO system (International Federation of Gynecology and Obstetrics) and the TNM system of the AJCC (American Joint Committee on Cancer)[8] .

Clinical classification requires a complete physical and gynaecological examination (including vaginal and rectal examinations and supraclavicular and inguinal lymph node assessment), radiological studies and additional procedures such as biopsy, conisation, cytoscopy and/or rectosigmoidoscopy[9] .

The FIGO system classifies cervical neoplasia into stages, stage I being when the invasive cancer is identified only microscopically, stage II when the carcinoma extends beyond the cervix but does not reach the pelvic wall, and may involve the vagina, but not in its lower third, stage III when the carcinoma extends to the pelvic wall and may involve the lower third of the vagina, showing no free space between the tumour and the pelvic wall on rectal examination, and stage IV when the carcinoma extends beyond the pelvis and involves the mucosa of adjacent organs (such as the bladder and rectum) and there is involvement of the pelvic and/or retroperitoneal lymph nodes[8,9,10] .

The AJCC SYSTEM, in turn, classifies cervical cancer based on the size of the primary tumour, the spread of the disease to regional lymph nodes and the spread of neoplastic cells to distant sites, characterising metastasis[9]

.

The most common treatments for cervical cancer are radiotherapy, combined with chemotherapy, and hysterectomy surgery[11] .

Radiotherapy is the most widely used loco-regional therapeutic modality for cervical cancer, fighting neoplastic cells through the penetration of radiation, which is created by the bombardment of accelerated electrons or gamma rays emitted by the radioactive material, thus preventing cell multiplication and/or determining apoptosis. It aims to eradicate the tumour causing minimal damage to adjacent tissues and is exclusively indicated in stages IIb, IIIa and IIIb(12) .

A pre-calculated dose of ionising radiation is applied to a volume of tissue that encompasses the tumour and is usually fractionated into daily doses, producing fast electrons that ionise the medium and create biochemical effects, such as the hydrolysis of water and the breaking of DNA strands, consequently promoting cell death, which occurs through the inactivation of vital cell systems. The tissue's response to radiation depends on a number of factors, such as the tumour's sensitivity to radiotherapy treatment, its location and oxygenation, the quality and quantity of the radiation, as well as the administration time(13) .

Two types of radiotherapy are used to treat cervical cancer: teletherapy and brachytherapy(12) .

Teletherapy consists of the irradiation of an ionising beam to the target region at a given distance, using radioactive sources of nuclear origin or linear accelerators, producing radiation through the acceleration of electrons(14) .

Brachytherapy consists of the delivery of 0 or Y radiation by an encapsulated source located a few centimetres from the tumour[12] . Another modality that has been widely used in clinical practice is high dose rate (HDR) brachytherapy, which aims to distribute a therapeutic dose prioritising the points of greatest neoplastic and proliferative activity, allowing for greater efficacy and a lower probability of complications[15] .

In advanced stages of cervical disease or to treat recurrence, chemotherapy can be administered concomitantly with radiotherapy, enhancing the effect of the treatment and increasing the patient's survival, despite the worsening of side effects. The most commonly used chemotherapy protocol for cervical cancer is cisplatin, which can be combined with other drugs such as carboplatin, paclitaxel, topotecan and gemcitabine[16] .

The effectiveness of treatment should be monitored by cytopathological examination, which has a sensitivity ranging from 28 to 51%, monitoring and detecting possible residual or recurrent neoplasms early on, allowing for immediate clinical and/or surgical intervention[9,17] .

The recommendations for the follow-up of women after radiotherapy, according to the AC Camargo Hospital Gynaecological Oncology Practice Manual, are clinical and cytopathological reassessments every 3-4 months for the first two years, with six-month intervals from the third to the fifth year of follow-up and annual return after 5 years[9] .

Radiotherapy is capable of promoting morphological changes, not only in neoplastic epithelial cells, but also in normal squamous and glandular epithelial cells, making it difficult to diagnose residual lesions, as these need to be well differentiated from reactive changes, avoiding the release of false-positive or false-negative results[17,18] .

In view of the importance of cytopathological analysis of the cervix after treatment and the difficulties of this investigation for pathological follow-up, the aim of this study is to report a series of eight cases of cytopathological evaluations after radiotherapy treatment for cervical cancer.

CHAPTER 2

Material and Methods

This is a descriptive case series study, which was approved by the Human Research Ethics Committee of the Tabosa de Almeida University Centre (Asces-Unita) under number 2.008.129.

Follow-up cytopathological collections and analyses were carried out using the conventional cytology technique in women with cervical cancer after radiotherapy treatment, assisted by an oncology centre in Pernambuco, between June and October 2017, after signing the Informed Consent Form (ICF).

To collect the cervical-vaginal material, the women first sat comfortably on the gynaecological table. The slide was labelled with the patient's initials, age and date of collection using an ordinary pencil on the matt side of the slide. The speculum was inserted into the vaginal canal in a vertical position and then rotated 90°, leaving it in a transverse position. The collection began at the ectocervix, with the longer end of the Ayre spatula inserted into the external orifice of the cervix and the mucosa scraped in a 360° rotating motion, exerting firm but gentle pressure without damaging the cervix. This material was then placed on the slide. To collect the endocervix, the brush was inserted into the cervical orifice, collecting the material by gently rotating it 360° and rolling it on the slide in a different direction to the material from the ectocervix. After arranging the material on the slide, cell fixation took place immediately by immersing the slide in a jar containing absolute liquid alcohol. For women who had undergone a total hysterectomy, the cytopathological material was only collected using Ayre's spatula, by scraping the vaginal dome.

The cervical-vaginal smears collected, after cell fixation for at least 30 minutes in absolute alcohol, were submitted to Papanicolau staining following the procedure below:

1. Immerse the slides in distilled water for 1 minute;
2. Haematoxylin staining for 15 seconds;
3. Hydration in a water bath;
4. Dehydration in absolute alcohol for 1 minute;
5. Dehydration in absolute alcohol for 2 minutes;
6. Coloured in Orange G6 with 5 dives;
7. Dehydration in absolute alcohol for 1 minute;
8. Dehydration in absolute alcohol for 2 minutes;
9. Staining in EA-36 for 4 minutes;

10. Dehydration in absolute alcohol for 1 minute;

11. Dehydration in absolute alcohol for 2 minutes;

12. Clear the bottom of the slide in xylene/alcohol for 2 minutes;

13. Dry the slide for 10 minutes in an exhaust hood.

After staining the smears, they were mounted with a mounting medium (varnish) and coverslip and left to dry for 1 day.

For microscopic analysis, the smears were assessed for the presence of post-radiation reaction effects in the squamous and/or glandular cells (cells increased in size, with the appearance of bizarre shapes, nuclei showing marked karyomegaly, with an irregular and sometimes degenerate shape and an increased nucleus/cytoplasm ratio[19]), indicating that the radiotherapy treatment had reached the target cells or, if the cells showed characteristics of premalignancy or malignancy (irregular chromatin distribution, coarse chromatin, changes in the shape and contour of the nucleus, hyperchromasia, cytoplasmic and nuclear polymorphisms[18]), indicating regression of the cervical cancer to low-grade squamous intraepithelial lesion (LSIL) or high-grade squamous intraepithelial lesion (HSIL) or recurrence and recurrence of invasive cervical cancer.

The sample was based on convenience, including all women seen during the proposed period, in any age group, with a diagnosis of cervical cancer confirmed by histopathology and who had undergone radiotherapy treatment.

Data was also collected from the medical records of women who underwent follow-up cytopathology during the proposed period, including: age group, histopathology result at diagnosis and treatment data.

CHAPTER 3

Case Reports and Results

Case 1

A.M.B.S., 65 years old, smoker, multiparous, histopathological examination showed undifferentiated squamous cell carcinoma. She underwent three sessions of chemotherapy with cisplatin and 5-fluorouracil, total hysterectomy and 28 sessions of teletherapy. The follow-up cytopathological examination was Negative for Intraepithelial Lesion and Malignancy (NLIM), showing a smear with a predominance of intermediate squamous epithelial cells, with slight reactive alterations (pseudoeosinophilia and polychromasia) and maintenance of the lactobacillary microbiota (Table 1; figure 1).

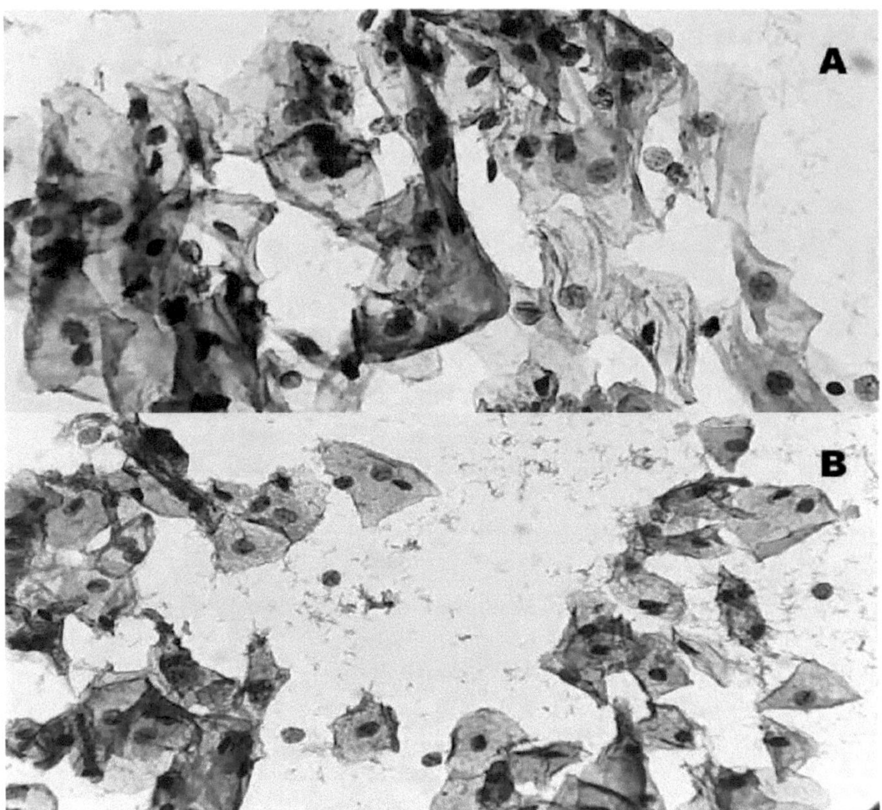

Figura 1: Negative for Intraepithelial Lesion and Malignancy. A: Predominance of intermediate squamous epithelial cells with slight reactive changes (polychromasia). B: Visualisation of bare nuclei and cytoplasmic debris, characterising the cytolysis of intermediate squamous epithelial cells by Lactobacillus spp. (400 X magnification).

Case 2

M.B.L., 36 years old, multiparous, histopathological diagnosis of squamous cell carcinoma. She underwent 26 sessions of teletherapy, 4 sessions of high dose rate (HDR) brachytherapy and 5 sessions of cisplatin. The cytopathological analysis revealed a NLIM result, the presence of superficial and intermediate squamous epithelial cells with marked reactive changes associated with radiation (polychromasia, cytoplasmic vacuolisation, cell gigantism, nuclear degeneration, nuclear pallor, anisokaryosis), metaplastic cells in various stages of maturation and coccoid microbiota (Table 1; figure 2).

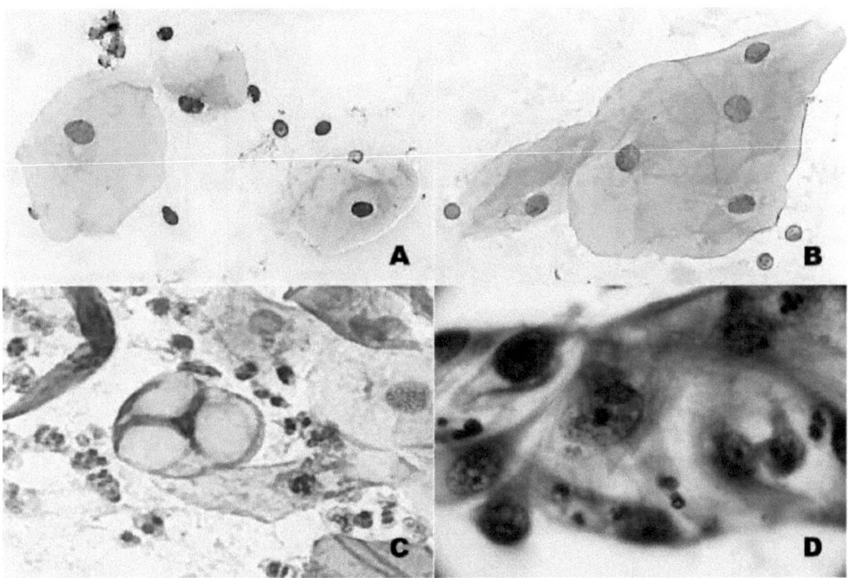

Figura 2: Benign Reactive Cell Changes Associated with Radiation. A: Intermediate squamous epithelial cell with cellular gigantism; B: Cellular gigantism and nuclear pallor; C: Cytoplasmic vacuolisation; D: Bizarre effects on metaplastic cells (400X magnification).

Case 3

M.M.C., 37 years old, multiparous, histopathological examination with result of undifferentiated squamous cell carcinoma. She underwent 28 sessions of teletherapy, 4 sessions of HDR brachytherapy and 3 sessions of cisplatin. Follow-up cytopathology revealed atrophy associated with inflammation, NLIM, predominance of parabasal squamous epithelial cells with moderate inflammatory changes (pseudoeosinophilia, polychromasia, nuclear pyknosis) and undetermined microbiology (Table 1; figure 3).

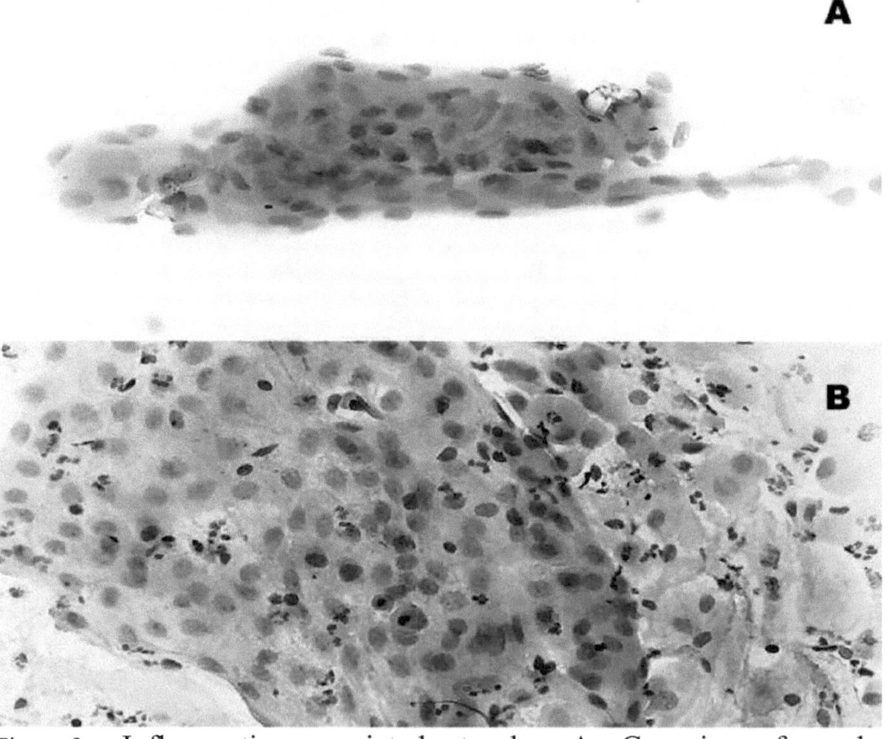

Figura 3: Inflammation-associated atrophy. A: Grouping of parabasal squamous epithelial cells with polychromasia. B: Predominance of

parabasal squamous epithelial cells showing inflammatory changes, such as polychromasia, pseudoeosinophilia and nuclear pyknosis, against a background of polymorphonuclear infiltrates (400 X magnification).

Case 4

M.A.R., 56 years old, multiparous, histopathology of moderately differentiated squamous cell carcinoma. She underwent 24 sessions of cisplatin, paclitaxel and carboplatin, 25 sessions of teletherapy and total hysterectomy. The patient reported abundant vaginal bleeding, which was also visualised on speculum examination. The material for cytopathological collection was vaginal and the result showed squamous cell carcinoma, with a predominance of parabasal squamous epithelial cells with marked nuclear (pleomorphism, hyperchromasia, coarse and irregularly distributed chromatin, anisokaryosis) and cytoplasmic (spindle and orangeophilic cells) alterations (Table 1; figure 4).

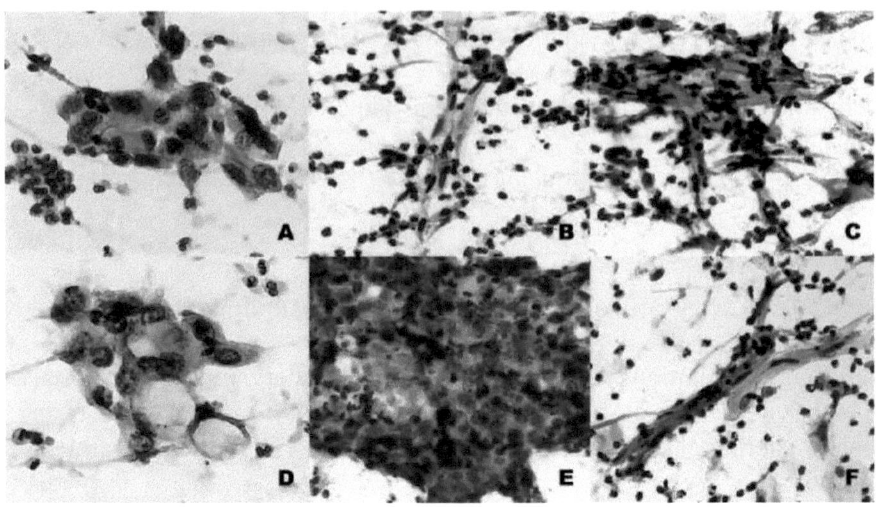

Figura 4: Squamous Cell Carcinoma. A: Parabasal squamous epithelial cells with karyomegaly, anisokaryosis, changes in the shape and contour of the nucleus and coarse, irregularly distributed chromatin; B: Pleomorphic, spindle-shaped squamous cells, orangeophilic cytoplasm, hyperchromatic nuclei and coarse, irregularly distributed chromatin; C: Spindle-shaped, orangeophilic cells and hyperchromatic nuclei; D: Parabasal squamous epithelial cells with altered nuclear contour and coarse, irregularly distributed chromatin; E: Syncytium of parabasal squamous epithelial cells with nuclear dyskaryosis; F: Orangeophilic, fusiform cells and hyperchromatic, elongated nuclei. (400X magnification)

Case 5

J.M.L., 41 years old, multiparous, histopathology of squamous cell carcinoma. She underwent 6 sessions of cisplatin and paclitaxel, 28 sessions of teletherapy and 4 sessions of HDR brachytherapy. The cytopathological examination was NLIM, showing superficial and intermediate squamous epithelial cells with moderate reactive changes associated with radiation (cell gigantism, cytoplasmic vacuolisation, nuclear degeneration, multinucleation, anisokaryosis), typical endocervical glandular cells, as well as metaplastic cells in various stages of reactive maturation (Table 1; figure 5).

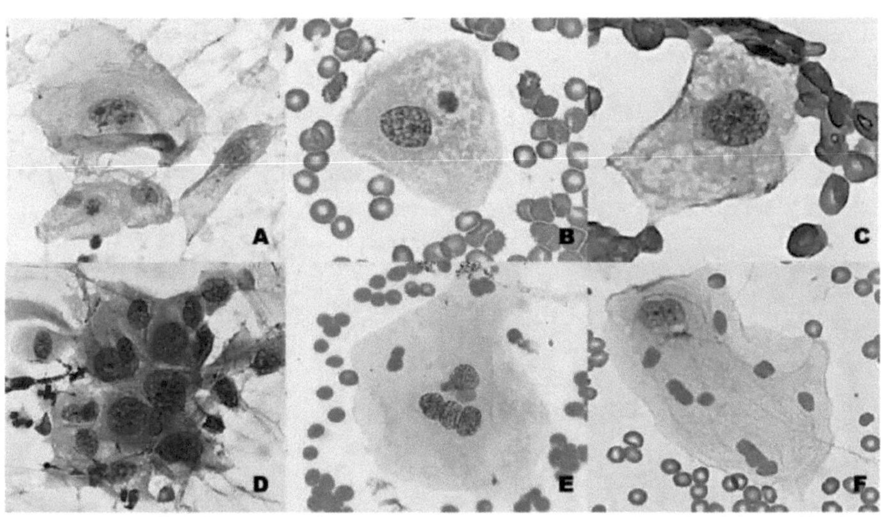

Figura 5: Benign Reactive Cell Alterations Associated with Radiation. A: Squamous epithelial cell with cellular gigantism and anisonucleosis; B: Cell showing nuclear degeneration; C: Cell with cytoplasmic vacuolisation and nuclear degeneration; D: Reactivity in metaplastic cells, with anisokaryosis and nucleoli; E: Multinucleated giant cell; F: Cellular gigantism and binucleation. (400X magnification)

Case 6

M.I.B.O., 66 years old, multiparous, histopathology showed moderately differentiated squamous cell carcinoma. She underwent 28 sessions of teletherapy and a total hysterectomy. Follow-up cytopathology was NLIM, but with slight inflammatory changes (pseudoeosinophilia), a predominance of intermediate squamous epithelial cells and a change in the microbiota with a predominance of supracytoplasmic bacilli suggestive of Gardnerella vaginalis and/or Mobiluncus sp. (Table 1; figure 6).

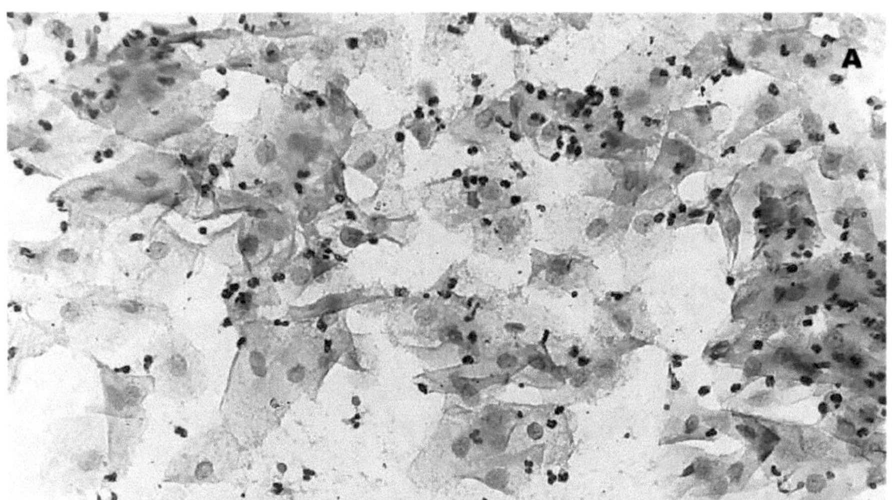

Figura 6: Inflammatory cytology. A: Predominance of intermediate squamous epithelial cells with slight reactive changes (polychromasia) and presence of supercytoplasmic bacilli (suggestive of Gardnerella vaginalis and/or Mobiluncus spp.) (400 X magnification).

Case 7

L.M.S., 47 years old, histopathology of well-differentiated squamous cell carcinoma. She underwent 28 sessions of teletherapy, 6 sessions of cisplatin and 4 sessions of HDR brachytherapy. The follow-up cytopathological analysis showed atrophy associated with inflammation, NLIM, a predominance of parabasal squamous epithelial cells showing moderate inflammatory changes (pseudoeosinophilia, polychromasia, cytoplasmic degeneration, karyorrhexis, nuclear pyknosis) and bacillary microbiota (Table 1; figure 7).

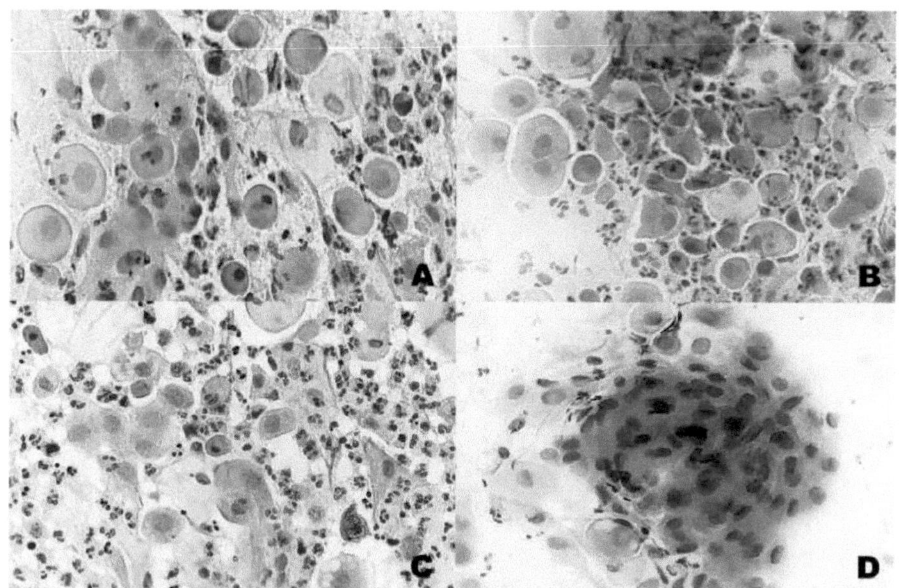

Figura 7: Inflammation-associated atrophy. A: Parabasal squamous epithelial cells amid a background of cell debris; B: Immature cells with benign reactive changes: nuclear pyknosis, pseudoeosinophilia and

polychromasia; C: Predominance of parabasal squamous epithelial cells amid a leucocytic infiltrate; D: Grouping of parabasal squamous epithelial cells (400X magnification).

Case 8

A.F.S., 27 years old, histopathological examination of undifferentiated squamous cell carcinoma. He underwent 3 sessions of cisplatin, 28 sessions of teletherapy and 4 sessions of HDR brachytherapy. The cytopathological examination showed rare superficial and intermediate squamous epithelial cells and numerous parabasal cells, the latter with reactive changes associated with radiation (cytoplasmic and nuclear vacuolisation, nuclear degeneration, anisokaryosis) and undetermined microbiota (Table 1; figure 8).

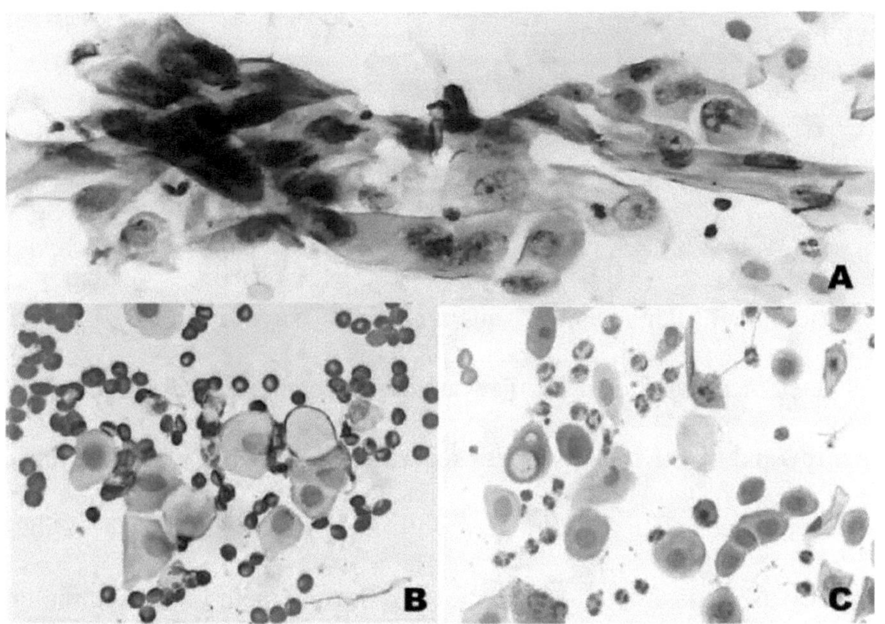

Figura 8: Benign Reactive Cell Changes Associated with Radiation. A: Squamous cells with degeneration and nuclear vacuolisation; B: Parabasal squamous epithelial cell with cytoplasmic vacuolisation; C: Benign reactive changes: cytoplasmic vacuolisation and polychromasia, as well as leukocyte infiltrate (400X magnification).

CHAPTER 4

Discussion

As for the profile of the women included in this study, there was a mean age of 46.87 years (standard deviation [SD] ± 26.87), 100% had a histopathological diagnosis of squamous cell carcinoma, 75% had 3 pregnancies or more and 62.5% had undergone concurrent chemotherapy, teletherapy and brachytherapy. With regard to the number of pregnancies, the data obtained in this study agree with the literature, which describes multiparity as a possible risk factor for the development of intraepithelial lesions and cervical cancer(20) .

Radiation can cause morphological and molecular changes in neoplastic and non-neoplastic cells through interference in messenger RNA synthesis, a decrease in protein production, inhibition of DNA synthesis and mitotic activity, as well as cytochemical changes, with denaturation of proteins and release of enzymes, with consequent destruction of cytoplasmic organelles(21,22) .

According to the literature, the cervical-vaginal smear is an excellent method for investigating and following up women undergoing radiotherapy for cervical cancer(17) . After the start of radiotherapy, for an average period of four to eight weeks, the cytopathological smear will show abundant necrotic material, with polymorphonuclear infiltrates and occasional malignant cells. Therefore, cytopathological examination is not indicated at this stage to assess persistent neoplasia. After this period, if sensitive to treatment, the malignant cells disappear and an atrophic cytological pattern is established. Benign reactive cell changes associated with radiation appear and are related to the acute and chronic phases after radiotherapy[21,23] .

In the present study, cytopathological follow-up ranged from 5 months to 10 years and 60.5% showed cellular alterations associated with radiation, with 3 cases (37.5%) having squamous cells showing benign reactive morphological alterations and 2 cases (25%) having an inflammatory atrophic pattern, which is defended in the literature as a finding induced by ionising radiation, since it promotes alterations in DNA, preventing the maturation process[17] .

With regard to the cytological findings caused by radiation in the cervical-vaginal smears evaluated, 3 cases (37.5%) showed cytoplasmic vacuolisation, nuclear degeneration and anisokaryosis, 2 cases (25%) cell gigantism and, only once, but in different cases (12.5%), nuclear pallor, multinucleation and nuclear vacuolisation.

Zannoni and Vellone[24] , evaluated the diagnostic accuracy of cytopathology in patients with cervical cancer after radiochemotherapy, finding 46% of smears with benign changes caused by radiochemotherapy, 20% with atrophy and 9% inflammation. The authors reported that nuclear and cytoplasmic enlargement, multinucleation, cytoplasmic vacuolisation and bizarre cell forms such as fibroblast-like, tadpole-like and anucleated cells were among the cellular alterations most related to radiation in the smears studied, corroborating most of the morphological alterations found in the present study.

According to various authors in the national and international literature, the main morphological findings induced by ionising radiation in cervical-vaginal smears are cytoplasmic enlargement, cytoplasmic vacuolisation, cytoplasmic degeneration, atrophy, cell gigantism, polychromasia, pleomorphism, karyomegaly, nuclear vacuolisation, nuclear degeneration, nuclear pallor, hyperchromasia, binucleation, multinucleation, karyorrhexis, nuclear pyknosis, anisokaryosis, multinucleated giant cells, leukocyte infiltrate, repair cells, multiple nucleoli and anisonucleosis(17,25) .

As radiation is associated with morphological changes in the cells of the cervix and vagina, cytopathological samples should be collected 3 to 4 months after radiotherapy to avoid the occurrence of unsatisfactory samples(23) . Wright et al(26) , evaluating the performance of liquid-based cytology using ThinPrep® in surveillance after primary or adjuvant irradiation in women with gynaecological neoplasms, concluded that the use of liquid-based cytology in the follow-up of women after radiotherapy is associated with a high rate of satisfactory samples, with only 2.7%(8/294) of tests described as unsatisfactory.

It was observed that in cases where radiation-induced morphological cellular alterations were revealed, the period between the end of treatment and follow-up cytopathology ranged from 5 to 16 months, with an average of 9 months. The acute effects of radiation tend to diminish gradually and, in most cases, morphological changes disappear from cervical-vaginal smears within 3-6 months of treatment. However, bizarre and enlarged cells can continue to appear in cytological smears for a period of years after treatment(27) .

The literature reports that the late effects of ionising radiation on the cervix and vagina promote the appearance of unusual benign squamous epithelial cells in cytopathological smears, such as cells with repair characteristics, large nuclei and macronuclei, multinucleated giant cells and highly vacuolised cells(27) .

All the cases in which the women underwent HDR brachytherapy also showed alterations post-radiation cellular reactions in follow-up cytopathology, justified by the extensive tissue trauma resulting from the insertion of applicators and probes, as well as the damage caused by the radiation itself, which is used at a high dose rate inside the tumour[28] .

The differential diagnosis of morphological characteristics associated with radiation includes repair processes, squamous intraepithelial lesions (SIL) and squamous cell carcinoma[17] . In this study, cases 2 and 5 showed cellular alterations that could be confused with those related to lesions and atypia, due to karyomegaly, slight nuclear hyperchromasia and "clear spaces" caused by nuclear degeneration, mimicking irregular chromatin distribution. However, nuclear alterations are always important for defining the diagnosis and, in these cases, they are not sufficient for the diagnosis of LIS, since no substantial increases in the nucleus/cytoplasm ratio were observed and the nuclei were pale and degenerated, without alterations in their shape and contour[19] .

In our series, one case of dyskaryosis by cytopathology, in cellular material from the vagina, revealed loco-regional recurrence. The clinical staging (FIGO) at diagnosis was IV A, as the carcinoma involved the bladder mucosa, justifying the recurrence found in this study[29] . Some authors have shown that post-radiotherapy recurrence rates increase according to tumour staging, with stage III and IV having the highest probability, with an incidence of 60-80% .[14,30]

Shield et al[31] , evaluating the role of cytopathology in the detection of recurrent cervical carcinoma after radiotherapy, revealed that the cytopathological diagnosis of carcinoma was present in 32.8% (23/70) of cases with recurrence confirmed by histopathology, at an average of 14.5 months after completion of radiotherapy, indicating that although follow-up cervical-vaginal cytopathology does not have high sensitivity, it is a reliable method for detecting recurrence and loco-regional recurrence, providing an early diagnosis of tumour reappearance or persistence, before the onset of clinical signs and symptoms.

Recurrent squamous cell carcinoma is diagnosed in the cytopathological smear when malignant cells are found after the conclusion of radiotherapy treatment, indicating radioresistance of the neoplastic cells, and it is possible to identify in the smear the presence of pleomorphic cells, hyperchromatic nuclei, thickening of the nuclear margins, coarse and irregularly distributed chromatin, increased nucleus/cytoplasm ratio, keratinisation of squamous cells, as well as morphological changes related to radiation.

[17,18]

In the study reported here, it was not possible to calculate the degree of sensitivity of follow-up cytopathology, since in the oncology service where the research was carried out, follow-up biopsy is not used routinely, and cytopathology is used as the method of choice, as well as the consensus recommendations of various authors in the literature[9, 17, 22 32] .

CHAPTER 5

References

1. José Alencar Gomes da Silva National Cancer Institute / INCA. Estimate 2018: Cancer Incidence in Brazil / José Alencar Gomes da Silva National Cancer Institute. Coordination of Prevention and Surveillance. Rio de Janeiro: INCA, 2017.

2. Campos ACC, Freitas-Júnior R, Poletto KQ, Goulart EF, Ribeiro LFJ, Paulinelli RR et al. Risk factors associated with cellular alterations induced by human papillomavirus in the uterine cervix. Rev Ciênc Méd. 2008; 17(3-6): 133-40.

3. Godoy IA, Fontana LC, Cordeiro EF, Khouri S, Strixino JF. Women's health: cytological and microbiological study of the genitourinary tract of patients at the UNIVAP supervised practice centre. Rev UNIVAP. 2014; 20(35): 5-14.

4. Becker DL, Brochier AW, Vaz CB, Oliveira JP, Santos MLV, Pilger DA et al. Correlation between genital infections and cervical cytopathological alterations in patients treated in the public health system of Porto Alegre. J Bras Doenças Sex Transm. 2011; 23(3): 116-9.

5. Silva ECA, Dias MP, Fernandes CK, Nogueira DS, Barros EJ, Mota RM et al. Knowledge of women aged 18 to 50 about the importance of the Pap test in the prevention of cervical cancer in the municipality of Turvânia-GO. Rev FMB.

2015; 8(4): 99-202.

6. Dias EG, Santos DDC, Dias ENF, Alves JCS, Soares LR. Socioeconomic profile and practice of cervical cancer screening among women in a health unit. Rev Saúde Desenvol. 2015; 7(4): 135-46.

7. Panobianco MS, Pimentel AV, Almeida AM, Oliveira ISB. Women diagnosed with advanced cancer of the cervix: coping with the disease and treatment. Rev Bras Cancerol. 2012; 58(3):517-23.

8. Rozenowicz RL, Santos RE, Campaner AB, Nadais RF, Rodrigues FFO, Rangel LRM et al. Comparative analysis of frequency, age distribution, body mass index (BMI) and tumour staging between adenocarcinoma and squamous cell carcinoma of the uterine cervix. Arq Med Hosp Fac Cienc Med Santa Casa São Paulo. 2006; 51(1): 10-3.

9. AC Camargo Hospital. Manual de condutas em ginecologia oncológica. 2ª ed. São Paulo: FAP; 2014.

10. Batista TP, Bezerra ALR, Martins MR, Carneiro VCG. What is the importance of the number of pelvic lymph nodes dissected for the locoregional staging of cervical cancer? Einstein. 2013; 11(4):451-5.

11. Zannoni GF, Vellone VG, Carbone A. Morphological effects of radiochemotherapy on cervical carcinoma: a morphological study of 50 cases of hysterectomy specimens affter neoadjuvant treatment. Int J

Gynecol Pathol. 2008; 27(2): 274-81.

12. Silveira CF, Regino PA, Soares MBO, Mendes LC, Elias TC, Silva SR. Quality of life and radiation toxicity in patients with gynecological and breast cancer. Esc Anna Nery. 2016; 20(4).

13. Fogaça JL, Vettorato MC, Camargo RF, Fernandes MAR. Analysis of radiometric parameters of radiotherapy procedures in cervical cancer. Rev Tekhne Logos. 2017; 8(4): 107-21.

14. Oliveira ACZ, Esteves SCB, Feijó LFA, Tagawa EK, Cunha MO. Interstitial brachytherapy for recurrences of cervical cancer after radiotherapy. Radiol Bras. 2005; 38(2): 117-20.

15. Bernardo BC, Lorenzato FRB, Figueiroa JN, Kitoko PM. Sexual dysfunction in patients with advanced cervical cancer undergoing exclusive radiotherapy. Rev Bras Ginecol Obstet. 2007; 29(2): 85-90.

16. Jorge LLR, Silva SR. Evaluation of the Quality of Life of Gynecological Cancer Patients Submitted to Antineoplastic Chemotherapy. Rev Latino- Am Enfermagem. 2010; 18(5): 849-55.

17. Padilha CML, Junior MLCA, Souza SAL. Cytopathologic evaluation of patients submitted to radiotherapy for uterine cervix cancer. Rev Assoc Med Bras. 2017; 63(4): 379-85.

18. Consolaro MEL, Maria-Engler SS. Clinical cervico-vaginal cytology:

text and atlas. 1ª ed. São Paulo: Roca; 2012.

19. Nayar R, Wilbur DC. The Bethesda system for reporting cervical cytology: definitions, criteria, and explanatory notes. 3ª ed. Springer; 2015.

20. Barroso MF, Gomes KRO, Andrade JX. Frequency of Pap smears in young women with an obstetric history in Teresina, Piauí, Brazil. Rev Panam Salud Publica. 2011; 29(3): 162-8.

21. Sharma M, Revannasiddaiah S, Gupta M, Seam RK, Gupta MK, Rastogi M. Can pure accelerated radiotherapy given as six fractions weekly be an option in locally advanced carcinoma cervix: results of a prospective randomised phase III trial. J Can Res Ther. 2016; 12(1): 1038.

22. Padilha CML, Feliciano GD, Filho LGP. Analysis of actinic effect after radiotherapy in the uterine cervix carcinomas. J Am Sci. 2005; 1(1): 1722.

23. Costa MOLP, Heráclio AS, Coelho AV, Acioly VL, Souza PR, Correia MT. Comparison of conventional Papanicolaou cytology samples with liquid-based cervical cytology samples from women in Pernambuco, Brazil. Braz J Med Biol Res. 2015; 48(9):831-8.

24. Zannoni GF, Vellone VG. Accuracy of papanicolaou smears in cervical cancer patients treated with radiochemotherapy followed by radical surgery. Am J Clin Pathol. 2008; 130: 787-94.

25. Powers CN. Radiation treatment effects in cervical cytology. Diagn Cytopathol. 1995; 13(1):75-80.

26. Wright JD, Herzog TJ, Mutch DG, Gibb RK, Rader JS, Davila RM, et al. Liquid-based cytology for the postirradiation surveillance of women with gynecologic malignancies. Gynecol Oncol. 2003; 91(1):134-8.

27. Shield PW. Chronic radiation effects: a correlative study of smears and from the cervix and vagina. Diagn Cytopathol. 1995; 13(2): 107-19.

28. Silva RMV, Pinezi JCD, Macedo LEA, Souza DN. The current situation of high-dose-rate brachytherapy in the cervix performed in Brazil. Radiol Bras. 2014; 47(3): 159-64.

29. Sadalla JC, Andrade JM, Genta MLND, Baracat EC. Cervical cancer: what's new? Rev Assoc Med Bras. 2015; 61(6): 536-42.

30. Mascarello KC, Silva NF, Piske MT, Viana KCG, Zandonade E, Amorim MHC. Sociodemographic and clinical profile of women with cervical cancer associated with initial staging. Rev Bras Cancerol. 2012; 58(3): 417-26.

31. Shield PW, Wright RG, Free K, Daunter B. The accuracy of cervicovaginal cytology in the detection of recurrent cervical carcinoma following radiotherapy. Gynecol Oncol. 1991; 41(3): 223-9.

32. Nanda K, McCrory DC, Myers ER, Bastian LA et al. Accuracy of the Papanicolaou test in screening for and follow-up of cervical cytologic abnormalities: a systematic review. Ann Intern Med. 2000; 132(10): 8109.

Table 1: Histopathological characteristics, treatments carried out and follow-up cytopathology results in women with cervical cancer after radiotherapy and/or chemotherapy.

	Idade	**Histopatologia**	**Início do tratamento**	**Quimioterapia**	**Teleterapia**	**Braquiterapia HDR**	**Cirurgia**	**Citopatologia de seguimento (Técnica convencional)**	**Material citopatologia**	**Resultado citopatologia**
Caso 1	65 anos	Carcinoma espinocelular indiferenciado *(Nov/2006)*	Julho/2007	3 sessões de cisplatina e 5-fluorouracil *(Jul/2007-*	50,4 Gy em 28 sessões *(Nov/2007-Dez/*	-	Histerectomia total *(Out/2007)*	Junho/2017	Cúpula vaginal	NLIM *Lactobacillus*

				Ago/2007)	*2007)*					
Caso 2	36 anos	Carcinoma espinocelular *(Nov/2016)*	Novembro/2016	5 sessões de cisplatina *(Jan/2017)*	26 sessões *(Nov/2016-Jan/2017)*	4 sessões de 700 cGy *(Jan/2017)*	-	Junho/2017	Ectocérvice / Endocérvice	ACBR associadas à radiação NLIM
Caso 3	37 anos	Carcinoma espinocelular indiferenciado *(Dez/2015)*	Dezembro/2015	3 sessões de cisplatina *(Jan/2016)*	50,4 Gy em 28 sessões *(Dez/2015-Fev/2016)*	4 sessões de 700 cGy *(Mar/2016-Abr/2016)*	-	Julho/2017	Ectocérvice / Endocérvice	Atrofia com inflamação NLIM

Caso 4	56 anos	Carcinoma espinocelular moderadamente diferenciado *(Out/2015)*	Novembro/2015	24 sessões de cisplatina, paclitaxel e carboplatina *(Nov/2015-Jun/2016)*	45 Gy em 25 sessões *(Jan/2016 - Fev/2016)*	-	Histerectomia total *(Abr/2015)*	Julho/2017	Vaginal	Carcinoma escamoso
Caso 5	41 anos	Carcinoma espinocelular *(Ago/2015)*	Dezembro/2015	6 sessões de cisplatina e paclitaxel *(Dez/2015-Fev/2016)*	50,4 Gy em 28 sessões *(Jan/2016 - Fev/2016)*	4 sessões de 700 cGy *(Mar/2016-Abr/2016)*	-	Agosto/2017	Ectocérvice / Endocérvice	ACBR associadas à radiação NLIM

Caso 6	66 anos	Carcinoma espinocelular moderadamente diferenciado *(Ago/2015)*	. Novembro/2015	-	50,5 Gy em 28 sessões (Nov - *Dez/2015)*	-	Histerectomia total *(Ago/2015)*	Setembro/2017	Cúpula vaginal	NLIM Citologia Inflamatória *Gardnerella vaginalis*
Caso 7	47 anos	Carcinoma espinocelular bem diferenciado *(Set/2014)*	Novembro/2014	6 sessões de cisplatina *(Nov/2014-Dez/2014)*	50,4 Gy em 28 sessões *(Nov/2014-Dez/2014)*	4 sessões de 700 cGy *(Jan/2015-Fev/2015)*	-	Outubro/2017	Ectocérvice / Endocérvice	Atrofia com inflamação NLIM

Caso 8	27 anos	Carcinoma espinocelular indiferenciado *(Dez/2016)*	Janeiro/2017	3 sessões de cisplatina *(Jan/2017)*	50,4 Gy em 28 sessões *(Jan/2017 - Mar/2017)*	4 sessões de 700 cGy *(Mar/2017)*	-	Outubro/2017	Ectocérvice / Endocérvice	ACBR associadas à radiação NLIM

NLIM: Negativo para Lesão Intraepitelial e Malignidade; **ACBR:** Alterações Celulares Benignas Reativas.

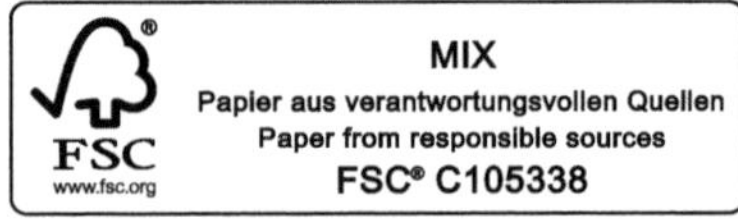

Printed by Books on Demand GmbH, Norderstedt / Germany